Welcoming Children from Sexual-Minority Families into Our Schools

by
Linda Leonard Lamme
and
Laurel A. Lamme

ISBN 0-87367-889-3
Copyright © 2003 by the Phi Delta Kappa Educational Foundation
Bloomington, Indiana

Table of Contents

Introduction 7

Understanding LGBT Families 9
   Types of Families 9
   What Can Educators Do? 14

**Sexual-Minority Families, the Community,
   and the Schools** 16
   Family Structures 17
   Adoption Issues 18
   Closeted and Out Families 20
   School Experiences of Children from
      LGBT Homes 22
   Students Who Are Closeted in School 25
   What Can Educators Do? 26

Creating LGBT-Friendly Schools 29
   Nondiscrimination Policies 30
   Faculty and Staff Training 32
   Gay-Straight Alliances 35
   Effective Counseling 37

Providing an LGBT-Inclusive Curriculum 39
   Countering Bias 40
   Challenging Heterosexism 42
   Connecting Curriculum to Resources 43

Resources 44

Introduction

Schools must be safe and supportive settings for all students. But students who are suspected of being gay or lesbian, or who have sexual-minority parents, often are targets of harassment. Epithets such as "dyke" and "fag" are common even in elementary schools. Students report verbal and physical abuse — and teachers who either ignore or participate in harassment.

In 2002 a student won a suit against the Washoe County, Nevada, school district and was awarded $451,000 on his claims of abuse and physical assault, which centered on his sexual orientation. The court ordered the district to establish new policies acknowledging a student's right to discuss sexual orientation as a matter of freedom of expression and required regular student and staff education about sexual harassment (Associated Press 2002). This suit will almost certainly not be the last brought against a school district that does not adequately protect its students.

Students especially hurt by such harassment are the children of lesbian, gay, bisexual, and transgender (LGBT) parents. This group experiences harassment to the same degree as do students who are thought to be gay, lesbian, or transgender themselves (Ray and

Gregory 2001). But often these students do not have access to programs or people who are prepared to meet their particular needs.

After our article on "Welcoming Children from Gay Families into Our Schools" was published in *Educational Leadership* (Lamme and Lamme 2001-2002), we received responses from grateful gay and lesbian parents, as well from resentful readers. Those who object to treating LGBT topics in schools usually ignore the fact that these efforts have little or nothing to do with sexual issues and everything to do with the lives and families of LGBT people and their children. One gay school principal wrote, "It amazes me that far too many people think, 'if we just ignore this, it will go away'; but then I also wonder why it does amaze me . . . people need to be educated, take time to come around . . . and with that time, eventually do." This man's conviction that, with education, the school climate will improve for sexual-minority parents and their children motivates us to continue to share information on how schools can become more welcoming to all children.

The first step is for educators to become more knowledgeable about LGBT families and the conditions under which they live. The second is to explore strategies for making the school climate more positive for these and other minority children. Third, we must examine the curriculum to make sure that it includes the history and presence of sexual-minority individuals and their contributions to society. Fourth, we must stress the need for teachers and counselors to have the resources and knowledge to support children of LGBT parents.

Understanding LGBT Families

According to the 2000 U.S. census, same-sex couples lived in 99.3% of the counties in America. Many of these households include children. In 1990 there were an estimated six million to 14 million children in the United States living with a lesbian, gay, bisexual, or transgender parent (Pellissier 2000; ACLU 1999; California Library 2000). With advancing reproductive technologies and more liberal adoption laws, more lesbian, gay, and transgender couples are deciding to have children than at any time in our history, causing a sharp rise in the number of LGBT families. Teachers and school administrators need to learn about these families in order to serve their children well.

Types of Families

There are many different kinds of sexual-minority families. Lesbian families have two moms, gay families have two dads, and transgender families have one or more parents who are transsexual or intersexual. Many LGBT families are "closeted," keeping their lifestyle a secret; others are "out," either open or partially open about their sexual orientation. Parents can be partnered, single, married, divorced, or partnered with another gay couple. LGBT parents have a more complex psychosocial environment than LGBT people without children, or than heterosexuals, because they have to integrate conflicting demands from both homosexual and heterosexual traditions (Bigner and Bozett 1990).

LGBT families can be rich or poor, religious or nonreligious, small or large, liberal or conservative, and biracial and multicultural (Spadola 2000). Children enter gay families in many ways — through birth, adoption, surrogate parenting, foster parenting, and artificial insemination. Regardless of their own eventual sexual orientation, these children become de facto members of the "gay" community, the term *gay* being shorthand for the entire scope of sexual-minority orientations. Whether or not their parents are active participants in gay-oriented events, they face a society that often is *homophobic* (fearing or disliking homosexuals) and *heterosexist* (focused only on heterosexual concerns or conduct).

School personnel need to become aware of both the unfortunate stereotypes that persist in our language and culture and the ongoing quest to redefine many of our unthinking assumptions. The word *family* itself has been used in a great deal of political maneuvering, often by those who seek to deny the existence of families that do not resemble a stereotypical, heterosexual ideal. Meanwhile, the children of LGBT parents themselves are undergoing a process of definition, without even a commonly accepted term to use for their own identity. "Children of lesbian, gay, bisexual, and transgendered parents" is cumbersome, if accurate. "Kids of gays" is shorter but excludes too many. "COLAGErs," from the name of the national organization, Children of Lesbians And Gays Everywhere, is not understood outside the community.

LGBT step-parents also are increasingly common. Children are born into heterosexual relationships before their mother or father partners with a person of the same sex, or an LGBT couple separates and the parents eventually establish new relationships (Erera and Fredriksen 1999). Children from these families have two issues with which to deal — the sexual orientation of one (or both) of their parents and the dynamics of divorce. Children of parents who separate amicably hear comments similar to those of the mom in *Daddy's Roommate* (Willhoite 1990) who says that "gay is just another way of loving." In other cases the straight parent may be hurt or offended and blame the gay parent for splitting up the family.

Children caught in the middle of any type of divorce need the support of school personnel, who should be careful not to take sides or malign either parent. Couples part, period. Whether heterosexual or homosexual dynamics are at work, such a parting profoundly affects the couple's children (Hennessy-Fiske 2001).

Not all sexual-minority individuals are gay men, lesbians, or bisexuals. Transgender, an umbrella term for people with various gender identities, includes transsexuals, who are born with sexual organs that differ from their gender identification. Many of these individuals go through a significant psychological and social transformation and considerable financial cost to obtain gender congruity. If they have children from a marriage prior to their change of gender, they typically lose custody; and their children have little or no support in attempting to understand the changed gender of their parent (Stuart 1991). If the transgender person subsequently marries, many judges will not grant custody to a couple that includes a transgender individual, even if it is the best situation for the children. *Transpeople*, as some call them, often are ignored by human rights groups focused on gay and lesbian issues (Garner 1999*b*). Regardless of custody issues, many children in our schools have transsexual parents because many transsexual individuals parent children before changing their identity or they adopt the children of their partners after changing their identity (Stuart 1991).

Intersexual people have genitals of both sexes. Somewhere between one in 500 and one in 1,000 have operations to obtain gender congruity. Intersexual people do not consider themselves gay, but their gender identities also can affect their family life and the lives of their children (Intersex Society of North America 2002).

Many U.S. families are "blended." Parents bring into a new relationship the children of a past one. There are "step-" fathers, mothers, brothers, and sisters. But our language does not offer easy ways to describe the relationship between a lesbian's children and her partner, her partner's children, or the rest of her partner's family, as it would if they were heterosexual. Children who may be legally able to use the last name of only one of their parents may then find their relationship with the other parent questioned. Also, with two parents of the same gender, children often use invented terminology for one parent. These affectionate terms may be unfamiliar to school personnel, but this does not mean that they do not indicate a deep and stable parental bond. As Laura Benkov, author of *Reinventing the Family*, writes, "The lack of cultural consensus about a term for lesbian and gay co-parents can be quite painful" (Benkov 1994, p. 172). For an article in the *Boston Globe*, Reilly Capps visited 335 lesbian and gay couples and their children gathered in Provincetown, Massachusetts, for an annual Family Week in the summer of 2002. He writes,

> Some people call themselves married, some call themselves partners. One dad is "daddy" while the other is "poppy." To their Cambodian daughters, Penny Bamford is "mommy" and Janine Cataldo is "makama," a variation on the Cambodian word for mom.... There's a new generation of gay people identifying themselves as moms and dads and this generation of kids has figured out their own language (for two moms or two dads). (Capps 2002, p. H1)

There is great interest on the part of the American public about gay families. The children's TV channel, Nickelodeon, ran a special on gay parenting on 18 June 2002, titled "My Family Is Different," which drew 976,000 adults from ages 18 to 49, the highest-ever ratings for the network's news specials (Advocate.com 2002). The show received heavy criticism from conservative groups, but it gave voice to important issues.

One child on the television program said, "You know, my family isn't all that different from any other family — we do chores, eat meals, go on vacations — we are pretty much the same as any other healthy family; we are pretty ordinary." That is one message that school personnel need to hear. Many LGBT families are pretty ordinary. Research indicates that children with lesbian and gay parents can develop psychologically, intellectually, behaviorally, and emotionally in positive directions and that the sexual orientation of parents is not an effective predictor of successful child development (Fitzgerald 1999). For the most part, family life for children who grow up in lesbian homes is similar to that experienced by children in heterosexual families (Tasker 1999).

What Can Educators Do?

An important step toward school improvement is for teachers and administrators to become comfortable interacting with sexual-minority individuals. Educators can visit bookstores and libraries to find books, magazines, and newspapers to learn more about LGBT families. (The Resources section of this fastback provides some starting points.) If educators also take time to make friends with LGBT individuals and ask them questions, they can discover a wealth of information firsthand. But having information does little good without developing a comfort level that will allow educators to interact with sexual-minority parents as easily as they interact with other parents.

Larger communities, in particular, also have LGBT-affirming churches, gay/lesbian community centers, and other organizations that welcome sexual-minority individuals and families. Educators can avail themselves of these organizations to obtain information, meet people, and grow comfortable interacting with individuals who are different from them.

Sexual-Minority Families, the Community, and the Schools

Many LGBT families actively participate alongside their "straight" (heterosexual) neighbors in child-oriented activities. Other families make it a point to take part in lesbian or gay social networks. Having children often paves the way for families to enjoy their straight and gay friends together instead of in segregated groups. Religious observance also serves to bring gay and straight families together in a larger community. Among the faith communities with long traditions of welcoming sexual-minority individuals into their congregations are the Unitarian Universalist Church, the United Church of Christ, and Reform Judaism. Metropolitan Community Church congregations are majority LGBT.

As much as there are ways in which LGBT families participate in the larger community, there also are challenges that sexual-minority families must face that set them apart. These challenges include the dynamics of family structure, adoption issues, legal matters related to partnering, being out or closeted, and prejudice related to having children outside a "traditional" family.

Family Structures

Many lesbian and gay couples choose to have commitment ceremonies, often conducted by clergy in churches and synagogues. Children may be included if a parent is one of the celebrants. Gay marriages are legally recognized in Denmark (since 1997), the Netherlands (since 1998), and Belgium (since 2003). On 12 July 2002 a three-judge Canadian court ruled that the Ontario government had to recognize same-sex marriages under the law (Kraus 2002). But, as of this writing, commitment ceremonies are not recognized as marriages in the United States.

Because lesbian and gay people cannot legally marry in the United States, children in their care are in an awkward, sometimes legally precarious situation. Their parents may feel that they must take various steps to ensure that a legal guardianship is in place should one parent die or become incapacitated. There have been cases in which children from lesbian and gay families have been taken away from a nonbiological parent who has raised them and have been given to relatives because their biological parent died. Such decisions cause a great deal of upheaval in both the parent's and the child's lives.

Lack of the availability of legal marriage has led some sexual-minority parents to make alternative arrangements. For example, a gay couple and a lesbian couple who are good friends may decide to form two "traditional" marriages — on paper — but raise the children in their lesbian or gay families. Such an alternative, if it works, can provide extended families for children, but heartbreak if they do not. Other lesbians and gay men choose to have children as single parents, usually with the support of family or friends.

School personnel should be aware of these extended and alternative family configurations so that all of a child's family members are treated with respect. "Respect" includes inviting partners, or co-parents, to parent-teacher conferences, informing them about the child's progress, and encouraging their participation in school functions.

The majority of LGBT households do operate very much like those of straight families. There are some cases where extended families, not approving of the "gay lifestyle," may be less than welcoming toward grandchildren; but usually such feelings soften with time. The problems these families experience are more often caused by societal discrimination and discriminatory laws, not their family configuration.

Adoption Issues

In many states lesbian, gay, and transgender adoption is impossible unless the prospective parents choose to lie about their sexuality. Florida bans any homosexual from adopting, while bans in Utah and Mississippi affect gay couples but not gay individuals (Perrin 2002).

Unlike the state of Florida, some states have moved to safeguard the interests of children with gay or lesbian parents. But the legalities of adoption by LGBT people vary greatly from state to state, and in many cases the laws are not clear. Twenty-one states now allow gay men and lesbians as individuals to adopt children; other states have ambiguous laws. Only 10 states grant same-sex couples the right to adopt (Human Rights Campaign 2003*b*). There also is evidence that social workers tend to be reluctant to place children in racial- or sexual-minority families (Ryan 2000). Up-to-date information on child custody and visitation laws affecting children of LGBT families can be found on the Human Rights Campaign website: www.hrc.org.

In February 2002 the American Academy of Pediatrics endorsed homosexual adoption, claiming that gay couples can provide the loving, stable, and emotionally healthy family life that children need. The academy pointed out that second-parent and co-parent adoptions are critical because of the following protections. Such adoption:

- Guarantees that in the event one parent dies or becomes incapacitated, the second parent would have his or her custody rights protected;
- Protects the rights of the second parent in the event the couple separates and ensures that children can benefit from child support from both parents;
- Allows children to be eligible for health insurance benefits from both parents;
- Gives both parents legal rights to consent for medical care; and
- Ensures children would be eligible for Social Security survivor benefits if one parent were to die.

Currently most children of lesbian and gay parents

do not have these rights and therefore suffer more than children of married parents in times of emergency, death of a parent, or separation of parents. The pressure on LGBT families in states that do not allow adoption by gay parents is enormous and is one reason that lesbians and gay men seek alternatives to adoption through surrogate parenting and artificial insemination (which also is denied to lesbians in many clinics).

Closeted and Out Families

Many LGBT parents live in fear that their employers will discover their sexual orientation or gender identity and they will lose their jobs. Parents who have children to support are especially vulnerable. Repressive laws and the lack of protective laws are the primary reasons that so many gay and lesbian adults are "in the closet," afraid to discuss anything involving their personal lives with co-workers or neighbors.

Living in the closet requires a large investment of time and energy that can sour relationships and deprive children of a carefree childhood. For example, partners may have to be careful not to express any affection in public. Most closeted families fabricate stories to explain their existence. One mother might be called "aunt," a designation that denies the parental closeness of a relationship. In many cases young children are not told about the nature of their parents' relationship so that they won't accidentally tell their playmates. When these children eventually find out, they can be devastated to discover that their parent is gay. They also may feel betrayed by the knowledge that was kept from them.

Closeted families are less likely to attend such public events as movies and ballgames as a family.

Children in closeted families may be afraid, often with reason, that if they betray their parents' sexuality, their parents could lose their job, their home, or be physically attacked. Depending on the custody laws of their state, which children are not always able to comprehend, they also may fear being taken away from their parents. These dangers, whether real or imagined, are a crushing burden for children of any age. Moreover, children from closeted families often may have to lie about their families, which can be embarrassing and upsetting. Pushing children to explain details only makes them feel pressed to lie more.

Sexual-minority families take various coming-out paths, and coming out can be long and involved. When families come out, at first they usually tell only accepting family members or friends, then gradually broaden the scope of their revelations (Lynch and Murray 2000). Safe spaces and supportive listeners in schools are vital supports for the many children in LGBT families that are closeted or in the process of coming out.

With few legal protections, out LGBT parents face being fired or evicted from their homes without justification. If their cars have rainbow flags or similar decals, they may be vandalized. LGBT people often face the impossible choice of remaining closeted and lying about themselves and their partners, or coming out and facing everything from subtle harassment to physical violence. Studies show that even mental health counselors (Patterson 2001) and psychiatrists (Crawford et al. 1999) discriminate against LGBT parents. Any of these conditions encountered by LGBT parents are bound to affect their children, if only indirectly.

When parents are open about their sexual orientation, their children are not forced to lie or hide but may encounter other problems. Besides possible discrimination and harassment, they may feel as if they are on display — representatives of their gay community — instead of being treated as individuals.

White LGBT parents face many problems, but matters can be worse for persons of color and ethnic minorities. Thus Latino, African-American, and Asian gay and lesbian parents (and individuals) tend to be more often closeted than do their white counterparts. They may identify more closely with their racial and ethnic communities than with the lesbian and gay community. There are also many multiracial lesbian and gay families. Children from these families face several sets of prejudices and need special support and recognition at school.

School Experiences of Children from LGBT Homes

Some children tease or harass any student who is "different" in some way: race, language, physical appearance — or a child of LGBT parents. In a study of the children of lesbians and gay parents in Australia, parents and children were surveyed and 75 of the children were interviewed to find out about their school experiences (Ray and Gregory 2001). The parents reported that their children's greatest concern in elementary through secondary school was feeling isolated or different. Lack of an inclusive curriculum and fear that their children would be bullied, teased, or discriminated against by a teacher concerned parents. Although the parents of primary school children reported few negative incidents, parents of middle and secondary school students reported many negative incidents.

The children were asked if they disclosed information about their parents' sexual orientation to fellow students. Most of the primary school students talked freely about their families, but by grade 3 they became less communicative. In grades 5 and 6 almost half of the students did not share information about their parents. Similarly, none of the younger children had been teased about their parents, but just under half of the older students had experienced being bullied with disparaging remarks and taunts. The children themselves often were labeled as gay. This bullying caused the children to feel a range of emotions from annoyance to extreme hurt. Most of the children ignored the bullying, recruited a friend to help them, or tried to explain about their family. Teachers did not take the harassment seriously.

To avoid harassment, more than one-third of the 12- to 16-year-olds did not disclose information about their parents. By the end of secondary school, more students, including those who had kept their "secret" for many years, were inclined to tell people. By that age their peers tended to be curious rather than antagonistic. Just under half of the students in grades 7 to 10 had been the victims of teasing or harassment that was related to the sexuality of their parents. That number dropped to 14% in the junior and senior years. When bullying did occur in middle and secondary school, it was harsher and included more severe physical abuse. Students reported being scared and trying to ignore the intimidation; boys sometimes tried fighting as a resolution. Older students did not talk with their parents about the harassment. They spent a lot of time avoiding being teased and victimized by trying to hide their parents' sexuality, using such strategies as not inviting friends over or setting up a false room in order to pretend that their parent's partner slept there. They lied or stretched the truth, sometimes carefully selecting one good friend so that they could reveal the truth about their family. Some actually joined in the teasing of other students to distract their peers. Older students were reluctant to go to teachers for help, and when they did, they found their responses inadequate. Students reported occasionally hearing teachers make homophobic remarks.

One interesting finding of this study was that children of lesbian and gay parents were bullied in school in the same proportions as students who were perceived to be gay — and at an earlier age. No extensive study of the school experiences of children of LGBT parents has been conducted recently in the United States. But there is no reason to believe that the results of this study cannot be generalized to U.S. schools. In general, Australia is viewed as a more accepting place for LGBT people than is the United States, and so these findings probably underrepresent the severity of U.S. problems. Many American LGBT parents cite as their reason for being closeted that they fear discrimination toward their child in school (Bliss and Harris 1998).

Students Who Are Closeted in School

Conflicting emotions about LGBT identity can cause stress within a family. Children can be closeted in school because they are fearful of repercussions if their classmates discover the sexual orientation or gender identity of their parents, or they can be closeted because their parents are closeted. Many children of LGBT parents have lost friends because of their parents' sexual orientation or gender identity, and so they already know that many people are hostile toward their family. Some children can find safe places in their neighborhoods, churches, playgroups, and social organizations. But school is a different story.

Children of LGBT parents may take precautionary steps to avoid confrontation. For example, by middle school, many children request that their parents take their rainbow flags or pink triangles off their cars so that their peers will not see them when they are dropped off and picked up at school.

Closeted children must constantly monitor their language so that they do not divulge that they have two dads or two moms. They may be reluctant to invite friends over to their house because the friends might notice gay or lesbian art, magazines, newspapers, or books. They may request that their parents lie about their relationship or that one of them not be evident at all.

What Can Educators Do?

Tapping local support can be valuable. For example, PFLAG (Parents, Families, and Friends of Lesbians and Gays) is a national organization that promotes the health and well-being of gay, lesbian, bisexual, and transgender persons and their families and friends. Local chapters of the organization function in many communities. And many PFLAG organizations become active in schools. The PFLAG website (www.pflag.org) lists 25 types of service that a local chapter (or similar group) can perform to help schools be more inclusive of LGBT materials in the curriculum and more accepting of LGBT people, whether students, parents, or educators. Any efforts that schools make to accommodate LGBT students also benefit children of LGBT parents. School personnel who wish to learn more about the LGBT community and to become advocates might join PFLAG.

The LGBT community is a subculture like that of any minority group, and many local media carry little news about minority groups in general. However, the *New York Times*, the *Boston Globe*, and other reputable city newspapers report positive news about LGBT people. Gay perspectives on topics in the media can be found in gay news sources. For example, *In the Life* is a nationally broadcast gay and lesbian television newsmagazine series, and *The Advocate* is a gay newsmagazine with national circulation. Educators who desire to become better informed about LGBT issues should visit a progressive bookstore for gay and lesbian newspapers and magazines. Many additional news sources are available online.

Discussing accurate, current, LGBT news items in class is a clear sign that school personnel are being aware and inclusive of children of LGBT parents. GLSEN (Gay Lesbian Straight Education Network; www.glsen.org) is an excellent source for news about LGBT people and schools. GLSEN defines itself as "the largest national network of parents, students, educators, and others ending discrimination based on sexual orientation and gender identity/expression in K-12 schools."

To help children of LGBT parents develop their own sense of community, educators might share with them information about COLAGE (Children of Lesbians and Gays Everywhere; www.colage.org). The stated mission of COLAGE is:

> To foster the growth of daughters and sons of lesbian, gay, bisexual and transgender parents of all racial, ethnic, and class backgrounds by providing education, support and community on local and international levels, to advocate for our rights and those of our families, and to promote acceptance and awareness that love makes a family.

Through COLAGE, children can participate in an online discussion group, find a pen pal who also has LGBT parents, and learn about Family Weeks and other gatherings of LGBT families. COLAGE is an exceptional resource for children of all ages.

Children in sexual-minority families also report that they appreciate participating in support groups at school. It is important to develop a gay-straight alliance in which students can join together to address homophobia and other forms of societal bias in their school environments. Such alliance groups offer a safe space for students to talk about their lives with others who will understand and accept them.

Finally, educators need to realize that, in spite of the fact that many children from LGBT families closet themselves at school, they almost uniformly report that there are advantages to growing up with lesbian or gay parents. Many such children enjoy feeling special and often are proud of being "different." They like being part of the gay community and socializing with other gay families, which leads to "talking about things we don't normally talk about," as some students will say. Older students realize that their upbringing has encouraged tolerance and an appreciation of difference. "I've been able to grow up with an open mind. And I bring that into the world and create more open minds.... I've been a support for gay kids," claimed one child of LGBT parents (Ray and Gregory 2001, p. 7). Certainly, as the United States becomes more multi-ethnic and diverse, people who can accept others and work together to solve problems become a great asset to our society.

Creating LGBT-Friendly Schools

The climate of a school includes the attitudes of teachers, staff, and students; physical surroundings and decorative items, such as posters or yearbooks; and other factors that combine, ideally, to make each student feel welcome and safe. If a school's climate is perceived to exclude certain students or pose emotional or physical dangers, it will interfere with these students' education.

A school district and individual schools can foster a welcoming climate for children of LGBT parents (and for LGBT students themselves) by taking several steps. For example, an overarching strategy might be to form a Safe Schools Coalition to determine the needs of each school, provide training and resources, and establish a support system within the school district. GLSEN can provide guidelines. Under the umbrella of a Safe Schools Coalition, a school district can create and enforce a nondiscrimination policy that includes sexual orientation and gender identity and expression; provides training for faculty, staff, and administrators; establishes a gay-straight alliance; and provides effective counseling services.

Nondiscrimination Policies

A school without a nondiscrimination policy that includes sexual orientation and gender identity and expression is not a safe place for children of LGBT parents. When LGBT faculty, staff, or administrators are afraid to be open about their sexual orientation because of job safety, they are hardly in a position to support or set a positive example for children from the LGBT community. Without such role models, fewer LGBT parents or students will feel safe being "out," and discrimination and harassment are more likely to be overlooked or even tolerated. A school without an inclusive nondiscrimination policy will have difficulty hiring qualified LGBT personnel.

According to the Safe Schools Coalition of Washington (Reis 2000), it is far easier to develop a warm and welcoming climate for children from gay families when there is diversity with regard to sexual orientation within the school administration, faculty, and staff. Schools seeking to be inclusive of all children should search for, hire, and retain a diverse staff. It also is important to establish explicitly protective, inclusive policies and collective bargaining agreements. Both children of LGBT parents and LGBT students claim that it is important to have sympathetic role models in their schools. The students in the Ray and Gregory study (2001) wished more faculty and staff members at their schools were open about their sexual orientation. They claimed that openly homosexual adults normalized the environment for them and their parents. A nondiscrimination policy that is enforced can go far toward wiping out the most common school problem for children of LGBT parents — fear of harassment and bullying.

School personnel must not let homophobia take root or tolerate intimidation of their students. "If there were no homophobia, I would be lying in bed thinking that I probably had one of the best days of my life" (Jack, grade 8, in Ray and Gregory 2001). Homophobia currently is a significant problem in our schools. It should be dealt with in the same firm manner as are racism and sexism, and teachers should be more determined to discipline bullies, according to children with gay and lesbian parents (Ray and Gregory 2001).

In survey studies all students report hearing homophobic remarks from peers, and one-third report hearing homophobic remarks from teachers (Massachusetts Governor's Commission 1993). LGBT students and children of LGBT parents are regularly threatened and ridiculed in school — the target of antigay violence and harassment. All school personnel need to join forces in refusing to tolerate any type of harassment, including homophobic epithets such as "faggot," "dyke," and "queer." School personnel who would never overlook racist or sexist terms are too often hesitant to address antigay words. When students in four San Francisco area schools heard homophobic remarks in school, 84% of the students reported never hearing an adult intervene (Pellissier 2000).

Hateful remarks should never be acceptable in any education environment. One study on violence in schools found that students who perpetuate violent acts often are students who have been verbally harassed by other students in their school (Bourke 2000). If for no other reason, we should acknowledge that violence begets violence, and we need to break the cycle.

Faculty and Staff Training

According to GLSEN, more than one-third of LGBT students do not feel comfortable talking with school staff about LGBT issues and therefore have no recourse should they encounter harassment or have personal problems. Children of LGBT parents experience homophobia in schools on a daily basis at an earlier age than do LGBT students. They often are reluctant to go to teachers for help because they find their teachers' responses inadequate (Ray and Gregory 2001). These findings demonstrate a need to provide diversity training for all school personnel and students, especially peer mediators and school counselors. There are many options for training, such as the resource module, "Tackling Gay Issues in School" (Mitchell 1999).

In addition to prohibiting negative language and actions, school personnel can counteract harassment and attempt to make schools more inviting for children from LGBT families. There are many ways to promote positive attitudes and atmospheres. The film, "It's Elementary: Talking About Gay Issues in School" (Chasnoff and Cohen 1996), features teachers at all grade levels discussing gay issues with their classes. Another vehicle for education is the touring "Love Makes a Family" photo-text exhibit, which includes photographs and texts of interviews with families of diverse racial, religious, cultural, and economic backgrounds with lesbian or gay parents, grandparents, or young adults.

Administrators need to keep faculty members, counselors, and other staff updated by distributing current research and publications on LGBT issues. They might consider subscribing to an LGBT family magazine, as well as publications about other minority groups. Such materials should be readily available in faculty lounges or school libraries. Diversity training, like effective training in other areas, should be ongoing and include periodic monitoring to determine its effect.

Communication is a key issue in developing a welcoming climate. Administrators, faculty, and staff can learn how to communicate in positive ways with LGBT families (Caspar and Schultz 1999). All written information, school signs, announcements to the press, student forms, and letters home should be inclusive. When addressing parents, for example, it is more inclusive to use the terms *spouse* or *partner*, instead of *husband* and *wife*. When communicating with gay families, educators should try to be sensitive to any special needs. If the family is divorced, it is best to send home two copies of everything, one for each side of the family with whom the child lives. If the child has two parents, there is no reason to ask, "Who is the 'real' parent?"; they are both real. If there is a legal reason for identifying the custodial parent, that is a different matter. But children in blended families, whether gay or straight, "belong" to both parents and likely will feel hurt if educators treat one parent as somehow less important. Educators can demonstrate that they understand the risks associated with disclosure if the family is closeted and should not ask students to discuss their parents in class unless they have talked about it with them individually — in private — beforehand (Caspar 1992).

Other ways that educators can visibly show their support include:

- Displaying gay-affirmative symbols, such as rainbow stickers, "Friends of Gays on Campus," and GLSEN logos, in offices and on school walls;
- Wearing pro-LGBT buttons and T-shirts;
- Displaying photographs of LGBT people and artwork by LGBT artists;
- Celebrating Gay Pride Month in the same manner as other "months," such as Black History Month or Women's History Month;
- Encouraging LGBT parents to speak at school or to volunteer in other ways, becoming visible in many roles; and
- Including LGBT parents and students in planning, decorating, and chaperoning school dances, an area in which many LGBT people have felt excluded in the past.

Planning occasions when diverse students can positively interact helps students get to know others who may not live in their neighborhood or take the same classes. Encouraging all students who wish to participate in athletic, musical, or artistic activities with their peers, regardless of traditional gender divisions in these areas, helps all students feel wanted and included. Other ways for students to create a diverse community include cooperative tutoring, inclusive student governments, and community action projects.

Gay-Straight Alliances

Most important at the middle and high school level is the establishment and support of a gay-straight alliance. An alliance support group provides a safe space in which students can share their personal experiences and learn techniques for dealing with harassment. Originally established for teenagers who are lesbian, gay, and bisexual, these organizations also provide advocacy for students who have LGBT parents. One student wrote, "The truth is, my father is the only reason I am involved. I fight for LGBT rights and equality because it is the right thing to do. I am not in the GSA just because I know and love someone who is gay, it is because I believe very strongly that no student should be unsafe at their school, simply because of who they are" (Parrish 2002). Support groups counter feelings of isolation, which can lead to depression and poor academic progress. Children from LGBT families, as well as LGBT students themselves, often report that the gay-straight alliance in their school is one of few places of safety (Ray and Gregory 2001).

The recent growth of gay-straight alliances (now in more than 1,000 schools nationwide) proves that they can be valuable resources for many students. Students can work with their peers, becoming proactive to end the victimization and harassment of students who are suspected to be gay or have LGBT parents. The GLSEN website contains information about starting and supporting gay-straight alliances. In addition to general support, such alliances can:

- Sponsor proms for LGBT students or help general prom committees to make proms pleasant occasions for all, not just straight couples.
- Provide a speakers bureau so that students may speak to classes or to the wider community about LGBT issues.
- Provide support for families whose LGBT loved ones commit suicide, run away, or encounter violence.
- Be advocates to the school board for nondiscrimination policies that include sexual orientation and gender identity.
- Write letters to local papers about safe-schools issues.
- Meet with school personnel, PTAs, and other parent groups as representatives of a diverse student population.
- Interact and cooperate with other minority groups.
- Provide peer facilitators for discussion groups on safe-schools issues.

In addition to gay-straight alliance groups for students, schools can structure staff-parent safe-schools groups. These groups can positively affect school climate by:

- Conducting research on the degree to which students experience verbal harassment and physical assaults;
- Monitoring schools' compliance with nondiscrimination policies; and
- Advocating legislation that protects LGBT students and students with LGBT parents.

School personnel also can show support by joining gay-friendly human rights organizations, such as Parents, Family and Friends of Lesbians and Gays (PFLAG) or the Human Rights Campaign (HRC), and by participating in community-based gay pride events.

Effective Counseling

Two groups of students need the attention of counselors. These groups include those students who are the target of harassment and discrimination and those who use homophobic language or act out in ways that bully or harass other students. The first group should have access to the best resources available for children of LGBT parents, including the resources of COLAGE and any support groups in the local community. Counselors also should be aware of their counterparts in private practice who have experience with LGBT families in the event that students need to be referred for counseling outside the school setting. Two LGBT resource magazines that can be useful for school counselors are *Alternative Parenting Magazine* (www.cybermale.com/magazines/alternativefamily.html) and *Gay Parent Magazine* (www.gayparentmag.com). These magazines contain references to other resources.

Effective counselors will help students of LGBT parents to interact with gay-friendly teachers, administrators, and other students. Feeling less isolated can make a significant difference in students' educational and social advancement. One experience that many children of gay parents share is surprise and pleasure at first meeting another child from a LGBT family. Although this will change as more LGBT people have children and do not feel the need to hide their orientation, it still happens seldom enough to be remarkable. Children from closeted families in particular may feel that they surely are the only one in their situation and can be especially grateful for the chance to talk with someone who understands.

Counselors must assure all students that gay families can be just as loving, cohesive, and stable as any straight family can be. Counselors should never "out" students, use them as gay family examples without their permission, or treat their family situation as unusual. If their parents are closeted, remind students that concealing the truth from a homophobic society does not mean that their parents are ashamed of themselves or their family.

Providing an LGBT-Inclusive Curriculum

Teachers often are unaware of the extent of bias in their curricula. Because the majority of teachers are white and middle-class, they often do not notice that the majority of stories and illustrations in textbooks are likewise about white and middle-class people. It all seems very ordinary to them. Models of racially and socioeconomically inclusive curricula exist to address this problem. While there is no doubt that black history should be covered throughout the year, having a Black History Month does ensure that teachers, who otherwise might not include minority history in the curriculum, will take notice. Many urban centers also have a Gay Pride Week or Gay Pride Month, but schools have been slower to recognize LGBT people and issues in the school curriculum. While curricula should include individuals who are gender nonconformists, in the early years of building a gay-friendly curriculum it helps to have a week or month in which the content can be emphasized and reinforced by outside news stories. Thus schools venturing into this sensitive arena for the first time can use Gay Pride Month to infuse, for example, famous LGBT people into the curriculum or to study important events in the history of LGBT people. Miller (1999) suggests a number of resources and strategies for bringing LGBT content into the classroom and infusing it into the curriculum.

Countering Bias

It is not sufficient for schools to reject harassment and violence. Students need to be taught acceptance of all people. An anti-bias curriculum should be established from early childhood onward. Students need information about all cultural groups. Teachers can mention gay issues when they discuss race and gender topics. And they can dispel gender stereotypes when such stereotypes appear in books, in the media, and in curricular materials. Children can be taught from early on to be critical readers for bias surrounding gender, race, social class, sexual orientation, and gender identity issues. Teachers should be able to identify the cultural assumptions behind classroom materials and discover what voices are being excluded so that they can then include those voices. Classroom lessons should include positive examples of many different types of families (adoptive, single parent, foster, etc.) as part of the curriculum. And teachers should affirm that all types of families can provide happy, successful home environments.

Older children from LGBT homes often claim that their exclusion from the curriculum begins in kindergarten (Ray and Gregory 2001). One man, reflecting on his school experiences, commented:

> Recently I saw for the first time a textbook that had gay parents in it, and I realized how radically it would have changed my life growing up — it would have wiped out the anxiety and suppression if I had seen this book when I was 10. The fact that I didn't have any friends whose mothers were lesbian didn't mean it didn't exist. I'm sure it did, even in Kentucky. You realize the drastic importance of having things public — talked about in school, for instance (Benkov 1994, p. 205).

Teachers also should pay attention when teaching about LGBT people. To teach about Oscar Wilde or Walt Whitman, for example, can be misleading without an understanding that both authors were gay. Silence is seldom "golden" when it means keeping silent about the sexual orientation of famous figures in history, literature, or the arts and sciences. Course content should include LGBT issues whenever it is appropriate and in context. Current news and other media coverage, especially from gay news sources, also present many opportunities to include gay and lesbian issues in classroom discussions.

Developing an LGBT-inclusive curriculum also involves identifying, challenging, and countering stereotypes of all sorts. Whether it involves language, appearance, gestures, or other features, stereotyping is simply that: typing. It means looking at "types," rather than "individuals," and it's the individuals who are important. Teachers and administrators may not be able to counter all of society's phobias or discriminatory laws, but they can give students a sense of the beauty and diversity of their LGBT cultural community.

Challenging Heterosexism

Simply stated, heterosexism is the presumption of heterosexuality. Because heterosexuality is the dominant sexual orientation, teachers and administrators often forget that not every student is straight or comes from a home with one male parent and one female parent. Many teachers have begun to be sensitized to blended and single-parent families, and the same must happen with regard to LGBT families.

Much of challenging heterosexism has to do with changing the language we use. For example, "Take this flyer home," rather than "Give this flyer to your mom," offers a neutral alternative, which is more suitable for students who may be from a home in which there is no "mom." Rather than referring to students as "boys and girls" — thereby potentially confusing gender identity matters — teachers can use nonsexist language: "students," "everyone." The separating of the sexes — "Boys line up here; girls over there" — often serves no purpose, and it may inadvertently contribute to compartmentalized or stereotypical thinking about gender roles. These are some first steps toward making classrooms places in which children are not deluged with expectations that they and their families should adhere to heterosexist gender roles.

Especially in elementary schools, teachers typically organize opportunities for children to honor their parents with homemade gifts, cards, or school performances on Mother's Day, Valentine's Day, and even Father's Day, which occurs after the school year has ended. These holidays can be stressful for children from single-parent or sexual-minority families. Students should be given every opportunity to make presents for or write about any parental figure they choose, without feeling singled out because they choose to do so.

Connecting Curriculum to Resources

It is impossible to offer a truly inclusive curriculum without a selection of good, recently published books on these topics in the school library. Children need to read both fiction and nonfiction about LGBT people and their children. When students see story characters like themselves in books, it normalizes their own family demographics and makes them feel less unusual. Unfortunately, there are not many high-quality books currently available, though more are published every year. But the books that do exist need to be in school and classroom libraries. Sometimes schools can obtain donations of books on these topics from LGBT alumni, from PFLAG, or from community human rights organizations.

Likewise there are some excellent and informative Internet resources that should be made available to students. Librarians should maintain resource lists of both traditional and online materials that describe families of all types. These can help all students who want to explore these topics. Some starting points are provided in the Resources section that follows.

Resources

These resources are helpful to learn more about the LGBT community, the school environment, and how to include LGBT studies in the curriculum.

Print

Benkov, L. *Reinventing the Family: The Emerging Story of Lesbian and Gay Parents*. New York: Crown, 1994.

Bigner, J., and Bozett, F. "Parenting by Gay Fathers." *Marriage & Family Review* 14 (Summer 1990): 155-75.

Bliss, G., and Harris, M. "Experiences of Gay and Lesbian Teachers and Parents with Coming Out in a School Setting." *Journal of Gay and Lesbian Social Services* 8 (1998): 13-28.

Bourke, D. "School Violence Study Is Chilling." *Gainesville Sun,* 28 October 2000.

Capps, R. "Family Week Gives P-Town New Slant on the 'Gay Lifestyle.'" *Boston Globe,* 15 August 2002, p. H1.

Caspar, V. "Breaking the Silence: Lesbian and Gay Parents and the Schools." *Teachers College Record* 94 (1992): 109-37.

Caspar, V., and Schulz, S. *Gay Parents/Straight Schools*. New York: Teachers College Press, 1999.

Chasnoff, D., and Cohen, H. "It's Elementary: Talking About Gay Issues in School." Videotape. San Francisco: Women's Educational Media, 1996.

Crawford, I.; McLeod, A.; Zamboni, B.; and Jordan, M. "Psychologists' Attitudes Toward Gay and Lesbian Parenting." *Professional Psychology, Research and Practice* 30 (1999): 394-402.

Edwards, A. "Let's Stop Ignoring Our Gay and Lesbian Youth." *Educational Leadership* 54 (April 1997): 68-70.

Erera, P.I., and Fredriksen, K. "Lesbian Stepfamilies: A Unique Family Structure." *Families in Society* 80 (May/June 1999): 263-71.

Fitzgerald, B. "Children of Lesbian and Gay Parents: A Review of the Literature." *Marriage & Family Review* 29 (1999): 57-76.

Hennessy-Fiske, M. "Molly Had Two Mommies (Divorce Among Gay Couples)." *The Advocate,* 11 September 2001, p. 9.

Howay, N., and Samuels, E. *Out of the Ordinary: Essays on Growing Up with Gay, Lesbian, and Transgender Parents.* New York: St. Martin's Press, 2000.

Jennings, P. *Becoming Visible: A Reader in Gay and Lesbian History for High School and College Students.* Boston: Alyson Press, 1994.

Kaiser, G.; Gillespie, P; Weston, K; and Pratt, M. *Love Makes a Family: Portraits of LGBT Parents and Their Families.* Amherst: University of Massachusetts Press, 1999.

Kraus, C. "Court Rules that Ontario Must Recognize Same-Sex Marriages." *New York Times,* 13 July 2002, Section 1, p. 9.

Lamme, L., and Lamme, L.A. "Welcoming Children from Gay Families into Our Schools." *Educational Leadership* 59 (December 2001/January 2002): 65-69.

Lynch, J.M., and Murray, K. "For the Love of the Children: The Coming Out Process for Lesbian and Gay Parents and Stepparents." *Journal of Homosexuality* 39 (April 2000): 1-24.

Massachusetts Governor's Commission on Gay and Lesbian Youth. *Making Schools Safe for Gay and Lesbian Youth.* Boston, 1993.

Miller, H. "Swimming with the Sharks." *The Reading Teacher* 52 (March 1999): 632-34.

Mitchell, L. *Tackling Gay Issues in School: A Resource Module*. GLSEN Connecticut and Planned Parenthood of Connecticut, 1999.

Patterson, C. "Families of the Lesbian Baby Boom: Maternal Mental Health and Child Adjustment." *Journal of Gay & Lesbian Psychotherapy* (Winter 2001): 91.

Perrin, E. "Technical Report: Coparent or Second-Parent Adoption by Same-Sex Parents." *Pediatrics* 109 (February 2002): 341-44.

Pollack, J. *Lesbian and Gay Families: Redefining Parenting in America*. New York: Scholastic, 1995.

Ray, V., and Gregory, R. "School Experiences of the Children of Lesbian and Gay Parents." *Family Matters* 59 (Winter 2001): 28-41.

Reis, B. *Safe Schools Report*. Seattle: Seattle-King County Department of Public Health, 2000.

Ryan, S. "Examining Social Workers' Placement Recommendations of Children with Adoptive Parents." *Journal of Contemporary Human Services* (September 2000): 517.

Stuart, E. *The Uninvited Dilemma: A Question of Gender*. Portland, Ore.: Metamorphosis Press, 1991.

Tasker, F. "Children in Lesbian-Led Families: A Review." *Clinical Child Psychology and Psychiatry* 4 (Spring 1999): 153-66.

"Times Will Begin Reporting Gay Couples' Ceremonies." *New York Times*, 18 August 2002, p. 30.

Willhoite, M. *Daddy's Roommate*. Boston: Alyson Publications, 1990.

Online

(Readers should be aware that online resources can be ephemeral. The following were current at press time. Also, online articles in archives sometimes cannot be accessed without paying a fee.)

ACLU Lesbian and Gay Rights Project. "ACLU Fact Sheet: Overview of Lesbian and Gay Parenting, Adoption and Foster Care." New York: American Civil Liberties Union, 6 April 1999. http://www.aclu.org/LesbianGayRights/LesbianGayRights.cfm?ID=92124C=104

Advocate.com. "Gay Parenting Special Scores Big Ratings for Nickelodeon." 2002. http://www.advocate.com/new_news.asp?ID=4781&sd=06/21/02

American Academy of Pediatrics. "AAP Says Children of Same-Sex Couples Deserve Two Legally Recognized Parents." 4 February 2002. http://www.aap.org/advocacy/archives/febsamesex.htm

Associated Press. "Endorsement of Gay Mentors at Big Brothers Big Sisters Causes Outcry." *Minneapolis St. Paul Star Tribune*, 16 August 2002. http://www.datalounge.com/datalounge/news/record.html?record=20141

California Library Fact Sheet. "Gay and Lesbian Adoptive Parents: Resources for Professionals and Parents." April 2000. http://www.calib.com/naic/pubs/f_gay.htm

Data Lounge. "Georgia Court Rejects Same-Sex Unions." 28 January 2002. http://www.datalounge.com/datalounge/news/record.html?record=18780

Data Lounge. "Huge Settlement Awarded in Harassment Case." 12 August 2002. http://www.datalounge.com/datalounge/news/record.html?record=20133

Garner, A. "Decreasing Homophobia in Schools." September 1999. http://www.familieslikemine.com/insight/ashley.html. (a)

Garner, A. "Learning about the Trans Community." July 1999. http://www.familieslikemine.com/insight/transphobia.html. (b)

Garner, A. "When Language Fails Our Families." July 1999. http://www.familieslikemine.com/insight/when_language_fails.html. (c)

Human Rights Campaign. "Domestic Partner Benefits." 2003. http://www.hrc.org/worknet/dp/index.asp

Human Rights Campaign. "Laws Affecting LGBT Families." 2003. http://www.hrc.org/familynet/chapter.asp?chapter=125

Intersex Society of North America. "Frequently Asked Questions." http://www.isna.org/faq/frequency.html

Parrish, M. "The S in GSA: Not Just Lip Service." 2002. www.glsen.org/templates/student/record.html?section=47&record=1388

Pellissier, H. "Nobody Does It Better." Salon.com. 2000. http://archive.salon.com/mwt/feature/2000/10/05/gay-parents/

Spadola, M. "Our House: A Very Real Documentary about Kids of Gay and Lesbian Parents." 2000. www.itvs.org/ourhouse

Helpful Websites

The Advocate.com. www.advocate.com

Alternative Family Magazine. www.cybermale.com/magazines/alternativefamily.html

American Civil Liberties Union. www.aclu.org

Chicago Free Press News. www.chicagofreepress.com/news/index.html

Children of Lesbians and Gays Everywhere (COLAGE). www.colage.org

Curriculum Resources for the P.E.R.S.O.N. Project: Books. www.youth.org/loco/PERSONProject/Resources/Books/list.html

Gay Lesbian Straight Education Network. www.glsen.org

Gay Parenting Magazine. www.gayparentmag.com

Human Rights Campaign. www.hrc.org

In the Life. http://www.inthelifetv.org

Love Makes a Family Exhibit. www.lovemakesafamily.org

Our House. www.itvs.org/ourhouse

Parents and Friends of Lesbians and Gays Everywhere (PFLAG). www.pflag.org

Recent Books Published by the Phi Delta Kappa Educational Foundation

Contextual Teaching and Learning
Susan Sears
Trade paperback. $10.95 (PDK members, $8.95)

Teacher Quality, Teaching Quality, and School Improvement
Leslie S. Kaplan and William A. Owings
Trade paperback. $12.95 (PDK members, $9.95)

Democracy and Intolerance: Christian School Curricula, School Choice, and Public Policy
Frances R.A. Paterson
Trade paperback. $19.95 (PDK members, $14.95)

Gifted Education: Promising Practices
Joan Franklin Smutny
Trade paperback. $17.95 (PDK members, $13.95)

Psychology of Success
Emery Stoops
Trade paperback. $14.95 (PDK members, $11.95)

Tutor Quest
Edward E. Gordon
Trade paperback. $10.95 (PDK members, $8.95)

Use Order Form on Next Page or Phone 1-800-766-1156

A processing charge is added to all orders.
Prices are subject to change without notice.
Complete online catalog at http://www.pdkintl.org

Order Form

SHIP TO:	
STREET	
CITY/STATE OR PROVINCE/ZIP OR POSTAL CODE	
DAYTIME PHONE NUMBER	PDK MEMBER ID NUMBER

QUANTITY	TITLE	PRICE

ORDERS MUST INCLUDE PROCESSING CHARGE

Total Merchandise	Processing Charge
Up to $50	$5
$50.01 to $100	$10
More than $100	$10 plus 5% of total

Special shipping available upon request.
Prices subject to change without notice.

SUBTOTAL	
Indiana residents add 6% Sales Tax	
PROCESSING CHARGE	
TOTAL	

☐ Payment Enclosed (check payable to Phi Delta Kappa International)

Bill my   ☐ VISA   ☐ MasterCard   ☐ American Express   ☐ Discover

ACCT #   DATE

/
EXP DATE   SIGNATURE

Mail or fax your order to: Phi Delta Kappa International,
P.O. Box 789, Bloomington, IN 47402-0789. USA
Fax: (812) 339-5556. Phone: (812) 339-1156

**For fastest service, phone 1-800-766-1156
and use your credit card.**